The Adrenal Reset Diet

Cure Adrenal Fatigue Naturally, Adrenal reset recipes, Adrenal reset program

By

Annabel Jacobs

Amazon Kindle Edition

The Adrenal Reset Diet

Copyright © 2014 by Annabel Jacobs

Introduction

Adrenal fatigue occurs when your adrenal glands do not function at the proper levels. It is often triggered by prolonged, intense stress. However it may also arise as the result of an infection. Especially one that affects the respiratory system, like pneumonia, influenza or bronchitis.

Adrenal fatigue causes symptoms that are similar to chronic fatigue syndrome; and is characterized by an overwhelming feeling of exhaustion that cannot be eased by rest or sleep. Often this is accompanied by a general feeling of malaise or un-wellness. Adrenal fatigue can also cause unwanted weight gain and high cortisol levels.

While adrenal fatigue affects literally millions of people worldwide, it has yet to be recognized as a distinct syndrome by conventional medicine.

HOW THIS BOOK WILL HELP YOU

This book help you assess whether your adrenal glands are tired or even crashed, and give you the best foods and methods to reset your body to full health. It will also help you lose any unwanted weight you have gained due to the chronic fatigue of the adrenal glands. The 7 Day Reset Program will guide you through specifically chosen meals to bring your energy back up and shed those unwanted pounds! I have also included 5 drink options that promote optimal adrenal gland health and recovery!

WHAT ARE THE ADRENAL GLANDS?

While the adrenal glands are small – only about three inches long and about 1.5 inches high – they are essential to healthy body functions. The most well known job of these small glands is to produce the hormone adrenaline. This is why they are most often talked about in terms of stress. Adrenal glands are triangle shaped, and are found atop each of your kidneys.

The adrenal glands consist of two parts, each of which has a distinct and important role in your body. These two parts are the **adrenal cortex** and the **adrenal medulla**. The **adrenal cortex** produces vital life hormones such as cortisol and aldosterone. Cortisol helps the body convert carbohydrates, fats, and proteins into energy. It also helps regulate blood pressure, which is necessary for a healthy cardiovascular system. The importance of cortisol in a healthy metabolism explains why adrenal fatigue can often lead to weight gain. The **adrenal cortex** also produces corticosterone, which works with cortisol to maintain a healthy immune system and suppress inflammatory reactions in your body. Aldosterone helps to regulate the salt and water ratios in your body, thereby maintaining healthy blood pressure. The adrenal cortex also releases small amounts of sex hormones (testosterone for men, and estrogen for women). **The adrenal medulla** – produces two different hormones, the best known of which is adrenaline. When your body senses stress, whether it is emotional or physical, your nervous system reacts by producing adrenaline. Adrenaline (also called epinephrine) helps your body cope with stress by sending more blood to the brain and muscles, and increasing your blood sugar levels. When you are suffering form adrenal fatigue, your body cannot adequately deal with stress. The second hormone produced by the **adrenal medulla** is noradrenaline, which also aids in stress reactions.

If you have low cortisol levels, you may become fatigued, because your body is not converting your food into energy the way it should be. You may also experience poor immune function, hypoglycaemia, and low blood pressure due to a slowed metabolism. An inability to deal with stress, and an increased sensitivity to your environment may be caused by low cortisol levels, and a poor functioning adrenal medulla. You may also have a higher tendency for allergies.

WHO IS AFFECTED BY ADRENAL FATIGUE?

Anyone can experience adrenal fatigue. Some people suffer from adrenal fatigue because of life style choices. This can include having a diet that is very heavy in processed foods, not having a healthy and consistent sleeping pattern, substance abuse, or an inability to decompress from high-pressure situations. Regular exposure to pollution, and the simple pressure of daily life can put real stress on the adrenal glands. Chronic or prolonged illness can also have a negative affect on these glands. Respiratory infections like pneumonia, or bronchitis may result in adrenal fatigue. It is also common for pregnant women to experience gestational adrenal fatigue.

MAJOR SYMPTOMS

Some of the common symptoms of adrenal fatigue include

• **Low blood sugar**- hypoglycemia often occurs in people suffering from adrenal fatigue because their metabolism slows down.

• **Low blood pressure**- this can often come along with dizziness, especially when waking up in the morning, or moving from a sitting to a standing position. This is due to irregularities with your body's ability to produce aldosterone.

• **Weight loss-changes** in weight may be due to metabolic problems.

• **Muscle weakness**- in a healthy body, challenging your muscles by lifting weights or running makes them stronger, as they break down and rebuild. In a person suffering from adrenal fatigue, the rebuilding of the muscle does not happen, just the break down. This can lead to muscular and joint weakness and pain.

Because any one of these symptoms can lead to serious complications, a timely diagnosis is crucial.

In cases of adrenal fatigue that are considered to be very severe, your adrenal glands may be so inactive that waking up in the morning, or going about your normal routine becomes difficult or impossible.

With severely decreased adrenal function, you may experience:

• **Weakness and fatigue -** particularly in the morning and afternoon hours

• **Increased allergies-** Often allergies to chemicals and foods will appear in people who were previously allergy free

• **Immune system becoming suppressed-** an increase in immune infections, and a slower recovery time are often a direct indicator of adrenal fatigue.

• **Depression-** feeling anxious, depressed, or unable to cope with daily stressors is an indicator that your adrenal glands may not be functioning properly.

• **Weight Gain -** without any obvious reason, especially in the belly and the thighs can be a sign of adrenal fatigue.

LESS OBVIOUS SYMPTOMS

Some symptoms of adrenal fatigue are less obvious. They include:

• **Hormone imbalances-** for women this can include an increase in PMS and symptoms of menopause. A decrease in libido is common in both men and women.

• **Cravings for fatty, sugary or salty foods-** craving fatty or sugary foods can be your body's way of coping with fatigue or lack of energy.

• **Autoimmune disorders-**cortisol plays an important role in the inflammatory process of the immune system. Problems with cortisol production can make it more difficult for your body to fight infection.

• **Skin issues-**an increase in acne, skin rashes, and a general loss of color in the face and hands are often linked to adrenal fatigue.

• **Decreased stress-**handling ability- feeling overwhelmed or unable to cope with daily life is often associated with exhausted adrenal glands

How Do I Test for Adrenal Fatigue?

Because adrenal fatigue is not currently recognized by conventional Western medicine, getting a proper diagnosis can be difficult. If you choose to go to a conventional doctor, you will likely have to take thyroid, cortisol, neurotransmitter, and total thyroxine tests, among others. If you are already suffering from adrenal fatigue, these testing methods can be exhausting as well as pricey. Luckily, if you fear that you may be suffering from adrenal fatigue, there is a quick simple test that you can do at home.

1 – To begin, stand facing a mirror, in a room that is darkened, for 15 seconds or more.

2 - Look into your mirror straight-on, and do not blink.

3 - Using a small flashlight, hold it at a point level with your eyes, about eight inches from the right eye.

4 - Move your light slowly around your head in the direction of your nose. Remember to stay eight inches away.

5 - Position your light at a 45 degree angle from your eye. Do not point it directly at your eye.

6 - Hold the light without moving, and count how many seconds your pupil maintains its contraction. You may count to as high as 20. Once your pupil loses its contraction or begins pulsing, stop counting.

7 - Repeat the same process on your other eye.

From 0 to 4 seconds = adrenal exhaustion

From five to 10 seconds = adrenal fatigue

From 11 to 19 seconds = adrenal dysfunction

20 seconds or more = proper adrenal function

This system for testing adrenal fatigue is called the Iris Contraction Test, and was first published in the 1920's. As can be seen above, people with healthy adrenal function should be able to maintain contracted pupils for at least 20 seconds. While this method is old, it is dependable and still used in alternative medicine today. This is a great way to quickly and non-invasively check your adrenal function.

FOODS FOR FATIGUE

Eating the right foods at the right times is very important to recovering from adrenal fatigue. While your diet will depend on your lifestyle and personal tastes, it is important to remember that good nutrition is the building block for recovery from adrenal fatigue. Some food groups will aid in your recovery, while others may impede it. While it may not be possible to completely change your diet, following these general guidelines will speed up your healing process.

FOODS TO AVOID

Sugar In those suffering from adrenal fatigue, limiting or totally avoiding sugar is crucial. When sugar reaches your blood stream, it creates a spike in insulin. While this may help your energy level right away, it is just a quick fix. Unfortunately, the high insulin levels are quickly cleared from your blood, so that burst of energy will crash just as quickly as it appeared. An excess of sugar also stimulates the release of cortisol, which in turn taxes the adrenal glands. The crash after eating sugar can lead to cravings, which can induce the consumption of stimulants like caffeine. Remember fruit contains fructose, which is a form of sugar. While generally a key component of a healthy diet, fruit should be limited during this 7 day Program to avoid insulin peaks and crashes. However, if taking fruit completely out of your diet is not feasible for you, try to stick with fruits that are low on the glycemic index. This includes apples, cherries, kiwi, and papaya.

Caffeine If you are suffering from adrenal fatigue, chances are you have been feeling the need to increase your coffee intake. Because one of the most predominant symptoms of this illness is a general feeling of exhaustion, it may seem that increasing your caffeine intake could be the answer. Unfortunately, excessive caffeine will only exacerbate the symptoms of chronic fatigue in the long run. Caffeine stimulates the part of your nervous system that tells your body you are in danger, causing it to go into fight or flight mode, which releases excess cortisol and adrenaline. The human body is excellent at adapting, and will quickly become accustomed to a certain level of caffeine. This will likely make you feel like you need to increase the amount you consume. However, increasing your coffee intake will only continue to increase your adrenal fatigue. While it may be tough at first, giving up that morning coffee will lead to more energy and happy adrenal glands! Herbal teas and ginseng are great substitutes for coffee in the morning!

FOODS TO EAT!

Your intake of vegetables is very important, and should be increased when trying to recover from adrenal fatigue. Veggies contain vitamins and minerals that help repair the adrenal tissue. During this diet you should eat between 6-8 servings of vegetables a day. Be aware that different cooking methods release different amounts and forms of nutrients. In general, it is best to eat veggies in their fresh, raw state whenever possible. If this is not an option, steaming is a great way to keep as much nutrients as possible in the vegetable. For optimal nutritional value, try and keep your vegetables as local and organic as you possibly can.

The Top 10 vegetables for treating adrenal fatigue are:

• **Kale** -this leafy green is a great source of vitamin C and calcium, both of which are crucial to stress management. Kale is also anti-inflammatory and an antioxidant, which will provide support to your taxed immune system.

• **Spinach** - this leafy green is rich in iron, magnesium, and vitamins C, B, and K. Magnesium is a natural mood stabilizer, and may help with anxiety or depression brought on by adrenal fatigue. Magnesium will also help with the joint pain and weakness that may come with adrenal fatigue.

• **Broccoli** - the high levels of Vitamin C found in broccoli help replace the low levels of this crucial nutrient that your adrenal glands need to produce cortisol.

• **Beetroot** - this delicious veggie is rich in vitamin C, vitamin A, iron, and fiber. All of which will help your recovering adrenal glands.

• **Peppers** -bell peppers are another great way to increase your Vitamin C intake without increasing your fructose intake.

• **Garlic** - garlic contains vitamin C and fiber to help replenish your adrenal glands. It also has been shown to help control blood pressure, and is a great way to healthfully season food.

• **Celery** - the healing properties of celery are well known in traditional medicine, and appear across the world in different remedies. For those suffering from adrenal fatigue, celery is useful for regulating blood pressure and as a vitamin C supplement.

• **Cucumber** - this veggie is high in vitamins C and B. Vitamin B is necessary for adrenal production, and provides energy in stressful times. Cucumbers are also anti-inflammatory.

• **Pumpkin** - Pumpkins are high in vitamins C and A, and fiber. Vitamin A will help with any skin issue brought on by adrenal fatigue, and high fiber is crucial for detoxing your adrenal glands.

• **Cauliflower** - cauliflower is an antioxidant and anti-inflammatory vegetable, so it provides support for your immune system. Cauliflower has also been shown to regulate blood pressure, and aid in proper cardiovascular function. This veggie is also great for those trying to detox from a high simple carbohydrate or processed food diet.

When recovering from adrenal fatigue, it is very important to keep your fructose intake as a low as possible. Insulin spikes due to a high sugar intake make it difficult for your body to recover normal adrenal function. That being said, in general fruits should be a mainstay in your diet as they provide vitamins, fiber, and antioxidants. Try to eat fruits that are low on the glycemic index, and rich in nutrients. The glycemic index is used to tell how high a specific food will raise the insulin level in your body, operating on a scale of 0 (no change) to 100 (pure glucose, major change in insulin levels). While recovering from adrenal fatigue, try and avoid any fruits with a glycemic index level over 70. Whenever possible buy organic and local fruits for optimal health benefits.

The Top 10 Fruits for Treating Adrenal Fatigue are:

- **Cherries-** Cherries rank lower on the glycemic index than most other fruits. They are a great source of antioxidants, and melatonin, and are anti-inflammatory. The antioxidants provide immune support, while the melatonin will help decrease the insomnia that often accompanies adrenal fatigue. The anti-inflammatory properties of cherries may diminish muscle and joint pain as well.

- **Apple-** Apples are also low on the glycemic index, as well as being low in calories. Apples are a good source of soluble fiber. Foods high in fiber help regulate your metabolism, keep you full longer, and promote digestive health.

- **Plum-** Plums are rich in antioxidants and potassium. The antioxidants provide aid in immune function, while potassium helps regulate blood pressure.

- **Kiwi-** The exotic kiwi is a delicious source of Vitamins E and C, fiber, potassium, and digestive enzymes. Vitamin E may help reduce any skin issues that have developed due to adrenal fatigue, while Vitamin C is necessary for a healthy immune system. The potassium found in kiwi is also beneficial for regulating blood pressure, another common issue for those suffering from adrenal fatigue.

- **Peach-**Peaches are known for being rich in Vitamins C, K, E, A. They are also a good source of fiber and magnesium. Among other benefits, the vitamins found in peaches aid in skin repair, immune support, and electrolyte balance. The magnesium that is found in this fruit is also helpful if adrenal fatigue has made you anxious or depressed.

- **Mango-** Mangos come in over 1,00 varieties around the world, but one thing that does not change from mango to mango is the health benefits of consuming them. Mangos are great sources of fiber and Vitamins A and C.

- **Strawberry-** Strawberries make an excellent snack for those suffering from adrenal fatigue. This fruit is packed with Vitamin C, fiber, and potassium. The anti-inflammatory agent in strawberries helps in immune function, and skin health.

- **Avocado-** While at first glance the avocado might look like a veggie, it is actually a fruit. Avocados are packed with the healthy fats needed to combat adrenal fatigue. They also aid in digestion, electrolyte balance, and immune system support.

- **Watermelon-**Watermelon has strong anti-inflammatory properties, is high in Vitamin C, and can help the kidneys detoxify. Watermelon is a diuretic, which means that it helps your kidneys process waste in a more efficient and quicker way. Watermelon is also good for promoting electrolyte balance within your body.

- **Pears-** Pears are high in fiber, and Vitamins C and K. They provide immune support, and help keep you feeling full. Very few people are allergic to pears, causing some doctors to call them hypoallergenic fruits. This means that almost anyone can enjoy the health benefits of pears without fear of a negative reaction.

Changing your diet can be an excellent place to start for treating adrenal fatigue. However, if your case is very severe, it may not be possible to get all of the necessary nutrients from food alone. In this case, adding herbal, vitamin, and mineral supplements to your diet can greatly aid in your recovery. Before taking supplements, it is always a good idea to check with your doctor, especially if you are already taking other medications. While herbal and mineral supplements can speed up your recovery, they should not be used as a replacement for a healthy diet.

The Top 10 Supplements for Treating Adrenal Fatigue are:

- **Magnesium**- Decreased levels of magnesium in the body is common in people suffering from adrenal fatigue. Magnesium helps your body deal with anxiety and depression. A lack of magnesium can lead to depression and fatigue, as well as muscle cramping and joint pain. Magnesium can be found in powder or capsule form at health food stores, or your local pharmacy.

- **Ashwaganda**- Ashwaganda is a plant originally from India that helps your body regain stress hormone balance. Ashwaganda is known as an adaptogen, meaning that it is supposed to regulate any imbalance within the body. It has been shown to be a calming agent, and reduce anxiety and depression. Ashwaganda usually comes in capsule form, and can be found at a health food store.

- **Licorice Root**- Licorice Root is a traditional remedy for low energy levels. It is a natural way to regain energy and vitality without increasing your caffeine intake. Unfortunately, this supplement has been shown to raise blood pressure, so be sure to speak with your doctor before beginning with this supplement.

- **Melatonin-**Melatonin is a great supplement for those suffering from sleeping problems. Melatonin is naturally produced in your body to regulate sleeping. If you suffer from insomnia, or inability to sleep deeply, melatonin is a great natural alternative to pharmaceutical sleep aides. Melatonin can be found at your local drugstore.

- **D-Ribose-** D-Ribose is a sugar, but it does not interact with your body in the same way fructose does. D-Ribose can be used to increase your energy level without caffeine. D-Ribose can be found at health food stores.

- **Vitamin C-**Vitamin C is necessary for proper adrenal gland function, as it helps produce cortisol and aldosterone. Supplementing your diet with Vitamin C will help with hormone production, and provide support to your immune system.

- **Vitamins B5, B6, B12-** All of these vitamins play important roles in your metabolism, which in turn helps your energy levels. B vitamins are also helpful in stress management. These vitamins can be found at your local drugstore.

- **Probiotics-** Every year more scientific studies appear linking emotional health to digestive health. Taking probiotics to aid in digestion and gut health can improve symptoms of depression and anxiety. Stage 3 of adrenal fatigue is often characterized by digestive problems, taking a probiotic supplement will also improve these symptoms.

- **Siberian Ginseng –** Siberian Ginseng functions as an adaptogen, and is very similar to Ashwaganda. It can be used as an alternative to caffeine to naturally increase energy and mental awareness. Just like Ashwaganda, Siberian Ginseng has been shown to increase blood pressure.

- **Omega 3-** Omega 3 fatty acid is one of the good fats to look for in your diet. Omega 3 reduces inflammation, which reduces the amount of cortisol your adrenal glands produce, and gives them time to recover.

While recovering from adrenal fatigue, you should also increase your intake of fiber. Fiber helps regulate sugar cravings and the release of sugar into the bloodstream. This helps stabilize your metabolism. Stabilizing your metabolism will in turn help stabilize your energy levels. Fiber is also important for detoxing from processed foods and sugars, which is necessary for a full recovery. Try to get your fiber from beans, lentils, vegetables and the supplement psyllium husk.

During the 7 Day Program you should only consume organic grass fed meats and wild caught fish. The pesticides and toxins regularly found in non-organic meat and fish will counter-act your detox process. Grass fed meat contains higher levels of healthy fats, but less overall calories. Healthy fat is important on this diet because it helps regulate metabolism. Organic meat is also free of the antibiotics found in conventional meat. Some research shows a connection between high exposure to antibiotics and a weakened immune system. Chances are that if you are suffering from adrenal fatigue, your immune system is already taxed. Wild fish is also higher in good fats, and less likely to have been exposed to harsh antibiotics or toxic pollution.

Although switching to exclusively wild, grass fed, and organic proteins may increase your food budget, it is well worth it. The goal of the 7 Day Program is to detoxify your body, and get you back to optimal health, which is priceless.

EXERCISE AND MEDITATION – WHAT'S YOUR FATIGUE LEVEL?

It is very important that you learn what stage of adrenal fatigue you are at. The treatments (and their effectiveness) for adrenal fatigue vary according to the severity of the case. Properly identifying your fatigue level is crucial to a complete and speedy recovery.

You must also do the right exercises when suffering from Adrenal Fatigue. Because muscle recovery does not happen as quickly (or at all) in people suffering from adrenal fatigue, it is important not to push yourself too hard. While daily exercise and physical activity are part of the foundation of a healthy body and healthy lifestyle, try to take it easy when dealing with this illness. If you push your body too hard at this time, you may see an increase in your symptoms. Outlined below is a guideline for exercising with adrenal fatigue, but first you have to understand what stage of the illness you are in.

Stage 1 – Stressed

You feel nervous as if about to go on stage, or speak in front of a large group of people. Often this begins as feeling stressed about a particular issue, but soon starts to spiral out of control. You may feel overly busy, have social anxiety, or a general feeling of being overwhelmed. Sleep problems like insomnia, or difficulty waking up in the morning may also begin to manifest in this stage.

Stage 2 – Wired but Tired

This is often described as a feeling of weakness paired with a strange sense of urgency. In stage 2, you will likely begin to feel some fatigue throughout the day, and an inability to sleep or clam down at night. At this phase, many people turn to caffeine in an effort to stay awake and aware at work. Unfortunately this will just exacerbate the problem, and move you into stage 3 more quickly.

Stage 3 - Crashed

This stage usually consists of pure exhaustion paired with digestive problems. Other symptoms of stage 3 include depression, weight loss, loss of sex drive, and general apathy. At this point, the hormonal changes in the body from a lack of cortisol, and imbalance of other hormones can begin to affect basically any part of the body.

Stage 1 – Perform 10 minute breathing style meditation & Stretches. Learning to relax through breathing and meditation can greatly help your adrenal fatigue symptoms. If you can learn to lower stress through these routines, you may be able to heal without going onto stage 2.

Stage 2 – Light weights & stretches. Light weight lifting, or resistance training can help to maintain muscle health without causing any damage or pain.

Stage 3 – Yoga or aerobics. Hatha yoga, which consists mostly of stretching and breathing, is low impact on your body. Try to stay away from high intensity programs like Bikram or hot yoga.

You may preform stage 1 & 2 exercise when at stage 3.

CHAPTER 2 – COMBAT WEIGHT GAIN!

Adrenal Fatigue can cause unstable cortisol rhythms. This leads to the storage of fat cells and we become more quickly fatigued. It can even lead to more serious issues like heart disease and diabetes.

CARB CYCLING

Carb cycling is a tool used to shed body fat. It can be very useful in managing cortisol levels, which is very helpful when trying to reset the Adrenal Glands. Cortisol levels are higher in the morning and lower in the evening. This process can be directly affected by protein and carbohydrate intake.

Carbohydrates should make up between 35 to 40 percent of your total calorie intake. Vegetables should be your primary carbohydrate source and make up half of your total food mass. Eating below 50 grams a day can block thyroid hormones and cause catabolism (muscle decay).

Most of your daily carbohydrate intake should be in the evening, because your muscles are more sensitive to insulin at night.

The simple method of carb cycling goes like this:

Morning – Low carb-Your first meal of the day should consist of mostly protein and healthy fats. Because your body metabolizes protein slowly, it sets you up for good energy and a healthy metabolism throughout the day.

Midday – Medium carb-Your midday meal should be an equal mix of carbohydrates and protein. This mix will give you the energy to make it through that mid-afternoon energy drop.

Evening – Medium/high carb-Your last meal of the day should be low protein and consist mostly of carbohydrates. This is because your metabolism will slow as you sleep, and you do not need the slow burning energy given by protein at this time.

Rotating your carbs like this allows you to shed body fat, while keeping your metabolism high. Since you repeat the cycle, you do not deprive yourself of carbs for too long which could potentially trigger the release of lipoprotein lipase.

By following this protocol you will be manipulating your blood sugar to achieve rapid weight loss.

CIRCADIAN REPAIR

The circadian human clock is the neurological system that signals the brain's pineal gland to produce the hormone melatonin, which aids in sleep. Poorly functioning adrenal glands can affect the circadian rhythm, which inhibits the ability to sleep at healthy times.

Light- Light striking your eyes is the most influential factor. When researchers invited volunteers into the laboratory and exposed them to light at intervals that were at odds with the outside world, the participants unconsciously reset their biological clocks to match the new light input. The circadian rhythm disturbances and sleep problems that affect up to 90% of blind people demonstrate the importance of light to sleep/wake patterns.

Time-As a person reads clocks, follows work and train schedules, and demands that the body remain alert for certain tasks and social events, there is cognitive pressure to stay on schedule.

Melatonin- Cells in the suprachiasmatic nucleus contain receptors for melatonin, a hormone produced in a predictable daily rhythm by the pineal gland, which is located deep in the brain between the two hemispheres. Levels of melatonin begin climbing after dark and ebb after dawn. The hormone induces drowsiness in some people, and scientists believe its daily light-sensitive cycles help keep the sleep/wake cycle on track.

It is imperative you follow these guidelines for proper circadian reset and weight loss:

1. **Get at least 7 hours of sleep per night**. This must include REM sleep. If you have trouble with this, try to get a sleep application on your mobile device to help make sure you are getting enough REM sleep.

2. **Consume 3mg of Melatonin 1 hour before bed**. This will help you sleep more soundly, and prevent the possibility of insomnia.

3. **Drink at least 4litres of water per day**. Hydration is key weight-loss and maintaining a healthy body.

CRAVINGS!

Most people think food cravings are their own fault due to a lack of discipline. The truth is it's just a chemical imbalance. You know you have food cravings when you have eaten a meal and still want something else to fix that urge. Craving sugary, or fatty foods is your body's way of coping with low energy. Because you are feeling fatigued, your body is looking for the quick energy spike induced by sugar, and other simple carbohydrates. However, while consuming these foods may make you feel better right away, in the long term they are just exacerbating your adrenal fatigue.

Many people also crave salt when suffering from adrenal fatigue. This is because your adrenal glands produce hormones that control the sodium balance in your body. If they are not able to do that job as efficiently as before, you will likely begin craving salt. Unlike the craving for sugar, for most people indulging in the salt craving is actually beneficial, and nothing to be too concerned about. Just be sure that you are satisfying that craving with high quality natural salt such as Himalayan Pink Salt, or Sea Salt. Try and avoid generic table salt, and as always steer clear of the of processed salty foods.

What does a healthy appetite feel like?

You should be hungry for healthy foods, and you should know how different foods affect your body. It is important to be compassionate with your body at this time, and understand that craving salt and sugar is not your fault. Snacking regularly will help you avoid sugar cravings, by keeping your metabolism going and providing a steady intake of energy.

HOW TO COMBAT CRAVINGS

Increase Fiber – Fiber slows the release of sugar in the body. You must have a steady release of energy into the body and fiber helps with this. You should consume soluble and insoluble forms of fiber. A great source of soluble fiber is blackberries. A great source of insoluble fiber is chia seeds. Fiber will also keep you feeling full for a longer amount of time. This may minimize your cravings.

Reduce Fructose – Fructose comes from high processed foods (high fructose corn syrup) and also regular sugar and fruits. The liver has to work extra hard to process fructose and this results in high blood sugar levels. Try to minimise fructose during the first part of the day. If you must consume fructose, try and get it from organic fruits. Fruits make an excellent dessert, and should be reserved for the later parts of the day.

7 Day Program

This is the 7 Day Program to kick-start your energy. The foods have specifically been chosen to promote proper adrenal function and reduce cortisol production. The meal plan virtually eliminates fructose, while still providing healthy treats to keep you from feeling like you are depriving yourself! It incorporates exercise to heal the circadian rhythm and get you on your way to losing weight! Simply follow this for 7 days to feel the results of proper hormonal function! Repeat again if pleased with results!

You do not need to count calories on this diet plan; the proportions of macronutrients have been specifically designed for the results we want.

Breakfast

Breakfast should be based around protein and healthy fats. This will keep you full and raise your metabolic rate. The idea of eating a high carbohydrate breakfast, full of bread and cereal does nothing but harm to your hormones and will leave you crashing at the end of the day, and a build-up of body fat at the end of the month!

Lunch

Lunch is best planned the day before, but this shouldn't be a problem as the program plans everything for you! Try to avoid fried food and sugary sauces as these will slow your energy production down and form toxic build up. Keeping your lunch a balance between complex carbohydrates and proteins allows for a steady metabolic release of energy throughout the entire day. The carbs will give you quick energy to get through the early afternoon, while the slow burning protein will keep you full and help avoid that 3pm slump.

Dinner

Dinner should be your highest carbohydrate meal. Because your metabolism slows at night while you sleep, there is no need to provide it with the slow burning protein needed to help you get through the beginning of the day. Eating a high carbohydrate dinner will also help you sleep better. Some of the recipes do not include many carbs at dinner so you are free to add a portion of your favorite carbohydrate source. Preferably choose a whole-grain, or vegetable source.

SNACKS/DRINKS

If you are not hungry then by all means omit the snacks, but if you are used to grazing then snacks are a great way to cram in some extra vitamins and minerals in the form of veggies! Snacks also keep your metabolism working, and prevent you from over eating during the meals. The snacks are also great way to satisfy cravings. Either consume the snack suggested in the program or swap it for a drink from the recipe section. The choice is yours!

DAY 1

Breakfast: Mini Chicken & Spring Onion Muffins

Morning Snack: Chinese Style Kale Chips

Lunch: Roast Butternut Squash Soup

Afternoon Snack: Adrenal Energy Bars

Dinner: Sticky Orange Chicken & Asian Slaw

Drinks: Choose from the list of Adrenal Reset Drinks, you may have up to 3 drinks a day.

Exercise: Choose from the list of Adrenal Reset Exercises depending on your stage.

DAY 2

Breakfast: Banana & Almond Butter Pancakes

Morning Snack: Crispy Sweet Potato Chips With Sage

Lunch: Japanese Style Burgers

Afternoon Snack: Adrenal Power Bomb!

Dinner: Spanish Style Clams

Drinks: Choose from the list of Adrenal Reset Drinks, you may have up to 3 drinks a day.

Exercise: Choose from the list of Adrenal Reset Exercises depending on your stage.

DAY 3

Breakfast: Ginger, Broad Bean & Turkey Burgers

Morning Snack: Zucchini & Pesto Roll Ups!

Lunch: Chicken Shawarma

Afternoon Snack: Chinese Style Kale Chips

Dinner: Comforting Chicken & Vegetable Soup

Drinks: Choose from the list of Adrenal Reset Drinks, you may have up to 3 drinks a day.

Exercise: Choose from the list of Adrenal Reset Exercises depending on your stage.

DAY 4

Breakfast: Toasted Coconut & Cinnamon Cereal

Morning Snack: Macadamia Hummus

Lunch: Roast Butternut Squash Soup

Afternoon Snack: Adrenal Energy Bars

Dinner: Dijon Crispy Salmon

Drinks: Choose from the list of Adrenal Reset Drinks, you may have up to 3 drinks a day.

Exercise: Choose from the list of Adrenal Reset Exercises depending on your stage.

DAY 5

Breakfast: Mini Chicken & Spring Onion Muffins

Morning Snack: Zucchini & Pesto Roll Ups!

Lunch: Sesame Seed Crusted Sea Bass & Cucumber Chilli Salad

Afternoon Snack: Macadamia Hummus

Dinner: Sticky Orange Chicken & Asian Slaw

Drinks: Choose from the list of Adrenal Reset Drinks, you may have up to 3 drinks a day.

Exercise: Choose from the list of Adrenal Reset Exercises depending on your stage.

DAY 6

Breakfast: Banana & Almond Butter Pancake

Morning Snack: Adrenal Energy Bars

Lunch: Japanese Style Burgers

Afternoon Snack: Crispy Sweet Potato Chips With Sage

Dinner: Spanish Style Clams

Drinks: Choose from the list of Adrenal Reset Drinks, you may have up to 3 drinks a day.

Exercise: Choose from the list of Adrenal Reset Exercises depending on your stage.

Day 7

Breakfast: Ginger, Broad Bean & Turkey Burgers

Morning Snack: Adrenal Power Bomb!

Lunch: Chicken Shawarma

Afternoon Snack: Macadamia Hummus

Dinner: Comforting Chicken & Vegetable Soup

Drinks: Choose from the list of Adrenal Reset Drinks, you may have up to 3 drinks a day.

Exercise: Choose from the list of Adrenal Reset Exercises depending on your stage.

ADRENAL RESET RECIPES

BREAKFAST

Mini Chicken & Spring Onion Muffins

Serves 2-3

Ingredients

3-4 boneless, skinless chicken thighs

½ crushed garlic clove

Salt and pepper to taste

¼ cup chosen hot sauce

¼ cup chopped spring onions

6 large eggs, whisked

3 tablespoon melted butter

Directions

1. Preheat oven to 425, and line muffin tins with parchment paper

2. Place chicken thighs on an oven roasting tray, and seasons with garlic, salt, and pepper. Roast for 35 minutes.

3. Put the cooked chicken into a bowl and shred into small pieces. Toss with the hot sauce, and set chicken aside.

4. In a bowl, whisk the eggs with the spring onions, salt and pepper.

5. Pour the egg mixture into parchment lined muffin tins, filling them approximately half way. Gently spoon about 1.5 0z of the cooked chicken, or enough to fill the cups.

6. Bake for 30 minutes or until the muffins rise and become golden. Enjoy!

Banana & Almond Butter Pancakes

Serves 2

Ingredients

3 Bananas

3 medium eggs

½ cup almond butter

2 teaspoons mixed spice

Directions

1. Heat skillet on medium.

2. Combine all ingredients in the blender and blend until smooth.

3. Grease skillet with coconut oil and pour the batter to make 3 inch pancakes.

4. Cook about 3 minutes each side

5. Serve with organic agave syrup and a squeeze of fresh lemon.

Ginger, Broad Bean & Turkey Burgers

Serves 2-3

Ingredients

1lb ground turkey

½ can broad beans

2 cloves garlic, crushed

1 teaspoon fresh ginger, grated

1 teaspoon fresh sage, finely chopped

1 teaspoon fresh rosemary, finely chopped

Salt and pepper to taste

1-2 tablespoons extra virgin olive oil

Directions

1. Pulse broad beans in a food processer until smooth. In a bowl combine the turkey, beans, garlic, ginger, sage, rosemary, salt and pepper.

2. Shape mixture into small burgers by molding them into a ball in the palm of your hand and then patting them down.

3. Heat the oil in a frying pan. Cook burgers in 2 batches.

4. Cook them for 4-5 minutes on each side. Enjoy!

Toasted Coconut & Cinnamon Cereal

Serves 2

Ingredients

3.5 cups unsweetened coconut flakes

2 tablespoons grass-fed butter

1.5 tablespoons cinnamon

4 tablespoon Swerve

Directions

1. Preheat oven to 340 F, and line a baking sheet with parchment paper

2. Put the coconut into a bowl.

3. Over a low heat melt the butter along with the cinnamon and Swerve.

4. Pour the mixture over the coconut and stir.

5. Spread the coconut over the lined baking sheet.

6. Bake for 5-6 minutes, stirring and flipping every few minutes to prevent burning.

7. Let it cool and serve with coconut milk.

LUNCH

Roast Butternut Squash Soup

Serves 2

Ingredients

1 large butternut squash

1 large onion, chopped

2 carrots, chopped

1 stick celery, chopped

4 tablespoons olive oil

2 teaspoons nutmeg

½ teaspoon cumin

3 cups chicken broth

Salt and pepper to taste

Directions

1. Preheat oven to 400 F. In a bowl combine the squash, oil, spices, salt and pepper. Mix together and place on a rimmed baking tray. Roast for 30-40 minutes or until soft.

2. Heat the remaining oil in a large pot and add the carrots, celery and onion. Cook gently for 10 minutes, or until vegetables are softened.

3. Add the squash to the pot along with the broth and cook for 15 minutes.

4. Using a liquidizer, blend until smooth. Enjoy!

Sesame Seed Crusted Sea Bass & Cucumber Chili Salad

Serves 1

Ingredients

7 ounces sea bass fillet, skinned

1 tablespoon sesame seeds

Salt and pepper to taste

1 tablespoon of grass fed butter

1 whole cucumber

½ red chili

Juice of 1 lime

½ red onion

Directions

1. Lightly season the sea bass fillet with salt and pepper. Lay the fillet on a bed of the sesame seeds, pressing down to ensure an even coating.

2. Melt the butter in a frying pan and cook the sea bass around 3 minutes each side and until golden brown.

3. For the salad: finely slice the onion and chili and place in bowl. Shave the cucumber over with a speed peeler. Add the lime juice, and salt and pepper to taste.

4. Serve the fish alongside the salad. Enjoy!

Japanese Style Burgers

Serves 2

Ingredients

1lb organic grass fed ground beef

1 onion

2 cloves garlic

1 egg

Salt and pepper

2 tablespoon Coconut oil

2 tablespoons tamari soy sauce

Directions

1. Grate the onion and garlic.

2. Mix the onion and garlic with the ground beef, egg, salt and pepper.

3. Heat the frying pan with coconut oil.

4. Split the mixture into 4 patties and pan fry each side for around 3 minutes.

5. Pour in the tamari soy sauce along with a splash of water, simmer for 2 minutes or until the burgers are coated in the sticky soy.

6. Enjoy!

Chicken Shawarma

Serves 2 -4

Ingredients

2lbs skinless chicken breasts cut into 1 inch pieces

¼ cup extra virgin olive oil

3 tablespoon freshly squeezed lemon juice

Salt and pepper to taste

½ teaspoon fresh thyme

2 teaspoons paprika

2 teaspoons cumin

2 teaspoons turmeric

2 teaspoons coriander powder

2 teaspoons cinnamon

Directions

1. Place the cut chicken into a bowl and combine the remaining ingredients and stir.

2. Let marinate for at least 2 hours.

3. Heat the grill and skewer the chicken on soaked bamboo skewers and grill for about 15 minutes or until cooked through.

4. Remove from grill and serve with hummus.

DINNER

Sticky Orange Chicken & Asian Slaw

Serves 1

Ingredients

1lb boneless, skinless chicken thighs cut into small pieces

3 tablespoons coconut oil

Juice of two oranges

Zest from one orange

1 teaspoon fresh ginger, minced

3 tablespoons tamari soy sauce

1 tablespoon chili & garlic sauce

4 scallions, chopped

1 cup white cabbage, shredded

1 cup red cabbage, shredded

½ cup spinach, shredded

Juice of two limes

Salt and pepper to taste

Directions

1. In a medium sized pot add the orange juice, zest, ginger, soy and chili sauce. Let it reduce down slowly.

2. In a frying pan heat the coconut oil over medium heat and add the chopped chicken. Cook until a golden brown crust has formed over the chicken.

3. Once the chicken is cooked, add to the pot with the sauce and stir though.

4. Serve in a bowl with the chopped scallions on top.

5. For the salad, combine the cabbages, scallions, spinach, lime juice, salt and pepper and mix in a bowl.

6. Serve the chicken on top of the salad, enjoy!

Spanish Style Clams

Serves 1

Ingredients

2lbs clams

1 tomato, diced

1 pinch saffron

1 cup fresh parsley, chopped

1 small bunch of thyme

1 clove garlic, crushed

Juice of half a lemon

Salt and pepper to taste

4 tablespoons extra-virgin olive oil

Directions

1. In a large, wide saucepan, heat the olive oil over high heat.

2. Add the garlic, tomato, saffron and thyme leaves and stir, until fragrant. No more than one minute.

3. Quickly add the clams, stir again and add the lid. Cook for 3 minutes or until clams are open.

4. Remove the lid and add the parsley, lemon juice, salt and pepper. (Go light on the salt as the clams are salty themselves).

5. Serve the clams with coconut flour bread. Enjoy!

Comforting Chicken & Vegetable Soup

Serves 4-6

Ingredients

6 cups chicken broth

Meat of whole chicken, diced

2 cloves garlic, crushed

1 large onion, diced

1 bay leaf

4 fresh tomatoes, sliced

2 small zucchini, thinly sliced

2 carrots, diced

Salt and pepper to taste

Directions

1. In a large pot, combine the broth, chicken, garlic, onion, bay leaf, and salt and pepper.

2. Bring the pot to the boil, reduce the heat to low and cover. Simmer for 2 hours.

3. Add the remaining ingredients and bring to a boil. Simmer for 15 minutes.

4. Serve in a bowl, Enjoy!

Dijon Crispy Salmon

Serves 4

Ingredients

1 ½ pound salmon fillet

2 garlic cloves, crushed

Juice of 1 lemon

4 tablespoons olive oil

1 tablespoon Dijon mustard

Handful fresh parsley

Handful fresh dill

1 tablespoon capers (in vinegar)

Salt and pepper to taste

Directions

1. Apart from the salmon, combine all the ingredients together in a small sauce pot.

2. Bring the sauce to a boil and simmer for 1 minute.

3. Place the salmon on a foil covered tray and spread the sauce generously over the salmon fillets.

4. Cook the salmon under the grill for around 10-12 minutes or until cooked.

5. Serve with a watercress salad or some baked sweet potato chips. Enjoy!

SNACKS

Chinese Style Kale Chips

Serves 2

Ingredients

A few handfuls of kale washed and dried

3 tablespoons extra-virgin olive oil

Sea salt to taste

1 teaspoon Chinese Five Spice

Directions

1. Preheat your oven to 300 degrees and slightly tear up the kale leaves to remove any big stems.

2. Toss the kale, olive oil and seasoning together in a bowl and sprinkle with the sea salt.

3. Lay the kale on a baking sheet (use two if there is a lot of kale) and cook for 12-15 minutes or until crisp.

Crispy Sweet Potato Chips With Sage

Serves 2

Ingredients

2 sweet potatoes, peeled

2 tablespoons extra-virgin olive oil

Sea salt to taste

A few fresh sage leaves

Directions

1. Pre heat oven to 350 degrees.

2. Using a mandolin, slice sweet potatoes to around 1/6 inch thick.

3. Grind or chop the sage and sea salt coarsely.

4. Mix the sweet potatoes in a bowl with the oil and herb mixture.

5. Place on a baking tray lined with greaseproof paper and the chips for 10 minutes.

6. After 10 minutes flip the chips and bake for 5 minutes.

7. Let them cool before serving. Enjoy!

Zucchini & Pesto Roll Ups!

Serves 2

Ingredients

2 large zucchini

About 12 cherry tomatoes

½ cup pesto (store bought or homemade)

Directions

1. Cut the ends off the zucchini. Using a vegetable speed peeler, peel off long strips off the zucchini.

2. Lay out a slice of the zucchini, spread a portion of pesto along the strip and place a cherry tomato near one end of the strip and start to roll. As you come to the end, spear the roll with a toothpick and place on a plate ready to eat! Make as much as you want!

Adrenal Power Bomb!

Serves 1

Ingredients

1 avocado

1/3 cup Greek yogurt

½ teaspoon cayenne pepper

Sea salt to taste

½ teaspoon garlic powder

Juice of half a lime

Directions

1. Slice the avocado in half, and remove the seed. Place the yogurt in the empty part of the avocado half, add the cayenne and garlic powder on top along with the salt.

2. Squeeze the lime juice over and enjoy!

Adrenal Energy Bars

Serves 2

Ingredients

¼ cup raw almonds

1 small banana

½ cup dried fruit

¼ cup flaxseeds

2 scoops vanilla whey protein

2 tablespoons arrowroot

½ cup almond flour

Directions

1. In a large bowl mash the banana and add the almond flour along with the arrowroot.

2. Add the rest of the ingredients and mix well.

3. Place the mixture onto a small greased baking sheet and press down to form a flat loaf.

4. Bake for around 30 minutes at 270 or until the edges are golden brown.

5. When finished, take out and cut the loaf into bar shapes. Best served slightly cool. Enjoy!

<u>Macadamia Hummus</u>

Serves 1

Ingredients

1 ½ cups macadamia nuts

Juice of 1 lemon

3 tablespoons olive oil

1 clove garlic

1 can chickpeas

Salt and pepper to taste

Directions

1. Place all the ingredients into a food processor and blend until smooth

2. Best served with crudities or alongside roast chicken!

DRINKS

The Berry Banger

Makes 3 servings

Ingredients

1 1/2 cup cashew milk

1/2 cup frozen raspberries

1/4 cup frozen cherries

1 tablespoon barley grass

Directions

1. Place all ingredients into your blender and blend to desired consistency. Enjoy!

Banana Butter Beauty

Makes 3 servings

Ingredients

1 1/2 cup cashew milk

1/2 peeled, frozen banana

2 tablespoons cashew butter

1 tablespoon barley grass

Directions

1. Place all ingredients into your blender and blend to desired consistency. Enjoy!

Reset & Thrive

Makes 2 servings

Ingredients

1 1/2 cup cashew milk

1 cup kale

1 cup baby spinach

1 handful frozen blueberries

1 tablespoon barley grass

1 cup ice

Directions

1. Place all ingredients into your blender and blend until smooth. Enjoy!

Citrus Sunshine

Makes 2 servings

Ingredients

Filtered water

1 Thinly sliced lemon

5 basil leaves

10 crushed strawberries

1 cup ice

Directions

1. Place all ingredients into your pitcher. Enjoy!

Orchard Delight

Makes 2 servings

Ingredients

2 large apples

Half of a peeled frozen banana

1 tablespoon cinnamon

A squeeze of lemon

1 tablespoon of honey

Directions

1. Place all ingredients into your juicer. Enjoy!

If you enjoyed this book, I would really appreciate it if you could leave me a positive review on Amazon.

I love getting feedback from my customers, and reviews on Amazon really do make a difference. I read all of my reviews and would appreciate your thoughts.

Thanks so much.

Annabel Jacobs